Dentists: What You Need to Know Before Choosing a Dentist

I0481849

By John Mitchsell

which the publisher or the original author of this work can be in any fashion deemed liable for any hardship or damages that may befall them after undertaking information described herein.

Additionally, the information in the following pages is intended only for informational purposes and should thus be thought of as universal. As befitting its nature, it is presented without assurance regarding its prolonged validity or interim quality. Trademarks that are mentioned are done without written consent and can in no way be considered an endorsement from the trademark holder.

Contents

Introduction..6

The Truth about Dentists All Being the Same.............. 8

How choosing the incorrect dentist could cost you time and money..11

Does your dentist provide an enjoyable overall experience?..17

Does your dentist understand your needs?...............22

Does your dentist offer a treatment plan for your review before starting a procedure?..........................25

Is your dentist up-to-date with the latest products and procedures?..27

Does your dentist allow a tour of the practice?..........34

Are dentists allowed to give nutrition and health recommendations?..36

Do dentists usually offer warranties on their treatments?... 37

How can your dentist remove mercury silver fillings safely for you?...40

What can you do as a patient before the amalgam removal procedure?.. 42

How to protect yourself during the appointment?.....44

What do you do after the procedure?........................ 46

What is sedation dentistry?....................................... 48

Cosmetic Dentistry.. 53

General Dentistry..54

Can teeth cleanings and exams be conducted by both General and Cosmetic Dentists?................................ 56

Are prices different between General and Cosmetics Dentists when it comes to the same procedures?...... 57

Which dentist would be best to replace a missing tooth? 58

Selecting an AACD specialist.......................................58

Why is an AACD accredited dentist beneficial?.......... 60

What is the accreditation process to become members of the AACD?.. 61

Shopping around for dental prices...............................62

What about dental insurance?.....................................64

Choosing dental insurance.. 68

Understand what the policy covers............................. 71

Dental tourism... 73

Why travel abroad for dental treatments?................. 74

The 10 Questions to Ask Your Dentist.........................79

Introduction

How often do you visit the dentist? Have you ever thought about your oral care and hygiene the same way you look at taking care of your body? If you are reading this book, chances are you are on the lookout for a good dentist but don't know where to begin. You may have been using one dentist for far too long, and you don't know what a good dentist actually is. There are plenty of reasons why you want to switch dentists. It could be your family dentist is retiring. It could be that you want to move away from your family dentist and use someone else. It could also be that you have moved to a new town and you are looking for a dentist closer to where you live. It could also be that your existing dentist does not offer the kinds of treatment you want or more comprehensive dental care that you require.

In this day and age, there are plenty of dentists out there advertising their businesses. Plus there is also the benefits of dental insurance which enables people to get better care for their teeth. The influx of dentists has also brought out the belief among potential patients that all dentists are the same.

Are all dentists the same? They are all graduates from a dental school, and they all needed to pass the state licensing and practicing licenses to become dentists. All these dentists also work in an office with the same kinds of equipment. Is there supposed to be a difference?

Hopefully in this short guide, you'll learn how to separate the good from the bad and choose the right dentist for you and your family

Thanks,

John Mitchsell

The Truth about Dentists All Being the Same

Let's begin with the very foundation of becoming a dentist- education. Not every dentist graduated first in their class even though all of them went through an accredited dental program and dental school. This does not mean that a good dentist is defined by their grades- it just means that graduating from a dental program does not necessarily qualify a dentist as a good one. By no means can grades measure skills- they only measure understanding of procedures, theories, studies, and facts.

However, you want a dentist that has graduated from an accredited program- that is first on your checklist. Next would be whether they are licensed or not. To be qualified to practice dentistry in your state, the dentist should pass a relatively easy test to get their practicing license. If your dentist is not licensed- do not use them.

Having a swanky office with state of the art facilities and equipment still does not mean that the dentist is a good dentist. It just means that she or he is well equipped with both the basic and extra tools needed to perform not just routine dental work but operations and surgeries as well.

Walk into any dental clinic or office today, and you'll be pleasantly surprised that most dental clinics are 'patient-centered' which means the dental office is equipped with a nice decor, friendly staff, free Wi-Fi, a coffee and tea area, etc. All these comforts are an addition to the clinic's services but do not necessarily reflect on the skills of the dentist. The area at which the dental clinic is located is also not an identification that the dentist is great. It only means that they have accomplished one of your needs which is ease of access.

The common perception is also that the best dentists can be found in Manhattan, NY but this is far from the truth. There are plenty of amazing dentists practicing all over the county that work in large and small towns, down the street, at family clinics and even in malls and rural areas. It is not the location but the skill of dentistry that these dentists possess that matter.

How choosing the incorrect dentist could cost you time and money

It is easy for a non-medical person to get carried away by what a medical person is saying all because we do not know what they are talking about and do not know what is the best treatment. That's why we give all our trust to the medical professionals that treat us.

But, you definitely want to know how someone without medical knowledge or dentistry knowledge knows if their dentist is worth their money? Here are a few pointers to look into to understand dentists and your money or insurance's worth:

Compare prices

It is only human nature to compare different services if you are having a hard time deciding which dentist to go with. If the dentist that you are using is more expensive than someone else in the area, you might want to start asking them to explain the difference in fees. Do not be afraid to ask because it is a perfectly reasonable thing to do- after all, you want to know what makes this dentist so different. It could be many reasons for a slightly higher price tag. It could be that they use different laboratories or it could be they use different materials or highest a bigger staff. Your dentist should give you some reason as to why this is the case without shutting you down by saying they have more experience or that they are more established.

Ask Questions

It is your tooth and your money. But in the midst of wanting to find out answers, be aware that you do not go overboard in questioning the integrity of the dentist and sound confrontational. You need to ask yourself why you need this and is the investment in dental care recommended by the dentist important to you in the long run. Would you be happy with basic dental care? Do you need to whiten your teeth often?

Your dentist would not want to recommend you dental work that is not useful or practical for you for the sake of getting more money. Oftentimes they would recommend what is best for your situation because, just like you, the dentist does not want to waste time dealing with cosmetic dental work when there are real issues they have to deal with other patients. When you understand the value of dental and oral care, you might not cringe so much at the cost.

Also, you can ask your dentist the length for a procedure such as for a crown (which usually takes five to seven months typically) or braces, which depends entirely on a person's mouth and teeth condition. Also, do the math with your dental insurance. Can you afford it?

Trust

Price is not the only deciding factor when it comes to picking a dentist. It also boils down to trust. Choosing a dentist is the same as choosing a gynecologist or a psychologist if you will. A huge emotional element is involved with it, apart from having someone else in your personal space. It is imperative to choose someone you feel comfortable with and above all, trust.

What is the best way to find a dentist you can trust? Word of mouth works best. Speaking to your colleagues, friends, and family to get recommendations for a dentist is a good start. Once you get a few recommendations, check their prices- a dentist's fees is just one part of the evaluation pie. You also want to have confidence and trust in the people you see when you walk into your dentist's clinic. Trust is important not only because it makes you feel comfortable but it also trust in the practice, knowing your dentist is capable of working and handling dental situations, recommending you the best form of treatment and also that they practice ethical dentistry such as sterilizing their instruments and equipment, staying updated with the dentist industry news, updates, drug information and so on.

You want your dentist to give you treatments and recommendations for your best interest in the long haul, not just ones that will bring in money to the clinic Prevention is, of course, better than spending a boatload of money on a dentist that does not do the job well.

Apart from going to your dentist for a good set of pearly whites, you also need to take care of your own teeth just so you do not reverse the efforts of the dentist and also waste the money you spent on getting your teeth fixed and cleaned. Brush every day, floss often and use a fluoride rinse.

Stop yourself and your kids from biting ice- ice is a crystal, and so it can hurt teeth enamel. When you push and bite both of these things, one of them breaks and in most cases, it is the ice, but sometimes, it can also be the tooth.

Does your dentist provide an enjoyable overall experience?

For plenty of us, going to the dentist is a nerve-wracking experience. Perhaps it may be the fact that we are opening our mouths wide and the ability to speak is hindered? Or maybe it's the fact that we don't know what to do while we are on the dental chair and all we're expecting is pain in the crevices of our teeth.

Whatever the reason, we know that despite the scary thoughts, regular dental checkups are vital for a healthy mind, body and of course, smile. Whether you need to go to the dentist for restorative procedures or cosmetic work such as teeth whitening or veneers your dental health is important.

So how can your dentist make the overall experience much more pleasant for patients, especially kids? Finding a friendly dentist that you trust, and one that you are comfortable with is essential, and one way to know if you'd be comfortable with your dentist is when you first meet the administration staff. The environment in the office should also be welcoming, immediately making you feel at ease.

Here are some ways dental clinics make the experience of visiting a dentist an enjoyable and pleasant experience:

Have fun

The layout and design of the dental practice have changed from a 'Doctor's office' with white walls and a melancholic atmosphere of doom and despair to an environment that is warm and welcoming. Dental clinics of today have moved away from the look and feel of a traditional medical office experience.

Employing fun people

The right people bring in the right atmosphere and plenty of dental clinics now strive to look for staff that are both knowledgeable but who are also people-oriented and have genuine concerns. A good sense of humor, empathy and a buoyant personality helps bring a sense of warmth to the place. The most crucial of all staff would be the one at the reception desk because they set the tone for the entire practice, setting a tone of positivity in both the practice as well as the mind of the patient.

Patients are still people

Dentists now help a patient ease into a dental chair by asking those things about themselves such as their favorite music, something about their family as well as their interests. A little small talk puts the patient at ease. Greeting each patient as though the dentist is very happy that they have arrived for their appointment with a big smile helps the dentist in getting the patient to be at ease but also can get the patient to speak a little bit more about their dental history. Grumpiness should be met with cheerfulness and friendliness. By being friendly, people will remember the dentist and the practice with inane cheerfulness.

A friendly environment

There is no law that says dental practices need to be white or any other color for that matter. A dental practice, especially one that serves children and toddlers can decorate their walls with pictures, colorful paintings, inspiring quotes and so on. There is no need to cover the entire wall with certificates of a dentist's accomplishments or scary clinical cases with diagrams that are hard to understand.

Playing Music

Playing music in a dental clinic gives off a charming and friendly feel. Some dentists even allow patients to choose their own music toplay during their appointment slots. This also creates a sense of belonging and puts the patient in a position of ease.

Decorating for every holiday

What better way to bring on the cheer of holiday spirit than with holiday decorations. Some dentists host a costume day for their staff, dress the dentist, put up Christmas trees of lights to amp up the cheer. At the end of the day, a fun practice is the best practice. A little bit of fun into the daily routine not only helps patients but also the dentist and the staff involved- it also creates a higher client retention rate for the clinic.

Does your dentist understand your needs?

It is important that your dentist understands your needs when it comes to dental treatment and care. It is also extremely important they listen to you and not just push you for treatment without taking into account if you can afford it if your work and life allows for this treatment and so on. You also are investing time and money into this which is why you need to make sure you feel safe, secure and confident in the hands of a qualified and experienced dentist.

How can you know if your dentist understands your needs? Here are five ways:

They are knowledgeable

Both the dentist and the staff are always ahead of the game and are continuously learning new techniques and ways to provide better treatment and care. A dental team must also be experts in dental assisting and hygiene and be equipped with a front desk that is on point with scheduling, financial information, and insurance information.

They explain your treatment

It may seem overwhelming when the dentist is explaining procedures and treatments for you. However, a dentist that understands your needs is a person that takes the time to explain what treatment is needed, the best options and also why you need it. The dentist must make you understand, and when you leave the clinic, you have the feeling of confidence knowing that the procedure is important and not completing it might lead to consequences you do not want.

They provide individualized care

Another way to know that your dentist understands your needs is by giving you individualized aftercare, for example, taking the time to make sure you understand insurance or cost-related information or the dentist checking up with you on your aftercare or encouraging you to call the dentist to give an update on your recovery or if you have any concerns or questions. Taking the time to see you not only as a patient but as a person, is a great way to know you can trust your dentist.

Does your dentist offer a treatment plan for your review before starting a procedure?

Dentist and in fact all medical practitioners have an ethical and legal obligation to obtain the informed and written consent of a patient before starting any kind of dental procedure or treatment.

When informing the patient, the discussion also needs to include information on costs and the patient's payment responsibilities. These estimates must include the cost of additional expenses for materials, lab fees if there are any as well as any other follow up treatment necessary such as a retentive appliance after an active orthodontic treatment or a crown following an endodontic therapy.

Provide exact costs and estimates

It is good practice for the dentist to provide the patient with the exact costs involved and if there will be any estimates. Providing the patient with a range of procedures following low and high costs will help and will also prevent the dentist from having to give an invoice that far exceeds the patient's budget. When a case is complex, dentists are also advised to provide costs for subsequent treatment due to unforeseen circumstances.

Answer questions

Allowing patients to ask questions only builds credibility and trust. A dentist should be open to any questions being asked and must commit to ensuring that the patient fully understands the treatment or procedure given to them and the costs involved. By being given the right answers, the patient has time to consider the various treatment options, and the dentist has done their part in ensuring all doubts and all concerns have been addressed.

Review the patient's financial arrangements

Once consent has been given by the patient, fees, and other financial arrangements should also be reviewed by the administration staff. Above all, the dentist must not only obtain consent, but it has to be informed consent. Only after this can treatment go on. In the event that the dentist has determined that there needs to be another treatment plan while the patient is in the chair, then the dentist must explain to the patient what the issue is and also the additional costs involved if any. A substitute decision maker must agree prior to the treatment continuing.

Is your dentist up-to-date with the

latest products and procedures?

How would a non-medical or non-dental person know if the dentist they are about to use is up-to-date with the latest 21st-century procedures and dental products?

This is a question asked by many. One of the first few things you can do as a patient is to read up and understand where dental care is today. If you have a friend who is a medical practitioner and knows these things, speaks to them. It is worthwhile to know what is happening in the dental industry before going to see a dentist.

That said there are also warning signs in the dental office itself that can tell you whether or not the dentist stays up to date. Here are some signs to look out for:

1. Your dental records are not requested by the Dental Clinic

Usually, the front desk staff of your new dentist's office will ask for your previous dental records as a baseline and also ask if you have any allergies. Dentists need to look for problems and changes in your teeth, and this can only be seen from x-rays. They usually see what's on the x-rays and check the patient's current teeth situations before suggesting any treatments or procedures. Some of these problems are very visible and having previous records such as X-rays are imperative in recognizing any developing issues.

A record of the past 6 months is usually requested either by the reception or the dentist themselves. Repeating X-rays too soon can cause unnecessary radiation exposure.

2. They're using old technology

If you have done your reading before going to see a dentist, you'd probably have a pretty good idea of what equipment is being used. Most dental offices in the USA use Digital X-Rays which gives the dentist a good diagnosis of cavities otherwise would not have been detected on traditional radiographs. When used as recommended by ADA, the digital X-ray has less radiation exposure than their film counterparts. It is always good to ask and check with your dentist on the kinds of equipment they would be using- even if you don't know what it does, your dentist should be able to answer them for you.

3. They're not careful about germs

Dentists are trained to ensure that there is no cross-contamination. This means that while they are with a patient, they have clean gloves on and they have a pack of sterilized equipment taken out freshly from the sterilizer. Dentists are so ingrained with the habit of being meticulous that it is second nature to them. However, if your dentist is touching the keyboard, answering their mobile phone and then poking about in your mouth without using fresh pair gloves- that is a big warning signal. Another question you may want to ask your dentist- Do you autoclaves the tools with heat sterilization, since most bacteria die only with heat? The dentist may think you're acting smart but then again, this is your right to ask and if a dentist explains to you the methods they use- that's great! If not, you have a problem with them.

4. No oral cancer screening is done

A compulsory check of your mouth for any signs of cancer should be done at an interval of every 6 months by your dentist. Oral cancer is connected to the Human Papilloma Virus (HPV), and while you may think that it is rare, the American Association for Cancer Research has reported that in the US alone this cancer has increased three times over the past two decades.

Your dentist will conduct an exam that involves looking for abnormal white or red patches of cells and lesions on the mucous membranes. The dentist will also feel the lymph nodes on your neck, check the insides of your cheeks, lift your tongue and inspect both sides, inspect your gum tissue and your throat as well.

5. Their gear is not made in the USA

This may be a hard question to ask, but if you really want to know, you can ask your dentist what labs they use for same-day dentistry. If you are getting crowns, or dental restorations, inlays, implants, dentures or orthodontic appliances, you can ask your dentist where it is manufactured. If you find that the dental practice is outsourcing lab work to a different country- this is a big warning signal too because it would mean that they care more about the bottom line than the quality of their dentistry and the patient's health.

What is your dentist's emergency policy?

If you have had work done on your teeth, another thing to ask your dentist is their emergency policy as well as their same-day appointment policy. Usually, dental clinics provide this information either on their website or most of the time on your appointment card so you can quickly refer to it when need be.

Also, find out how to contact your dentist if you need urgent care or treatment, and you require it after normal office hours. Dentists typically have an emergency plan for cases like this, and their patients can contact them or make arrangements with other dentists nearby.

Does your dentist allow a tour of the practice?

Quite often, getting a tour of the dental practice can calm a person down and allow them to overcome dental anxiety. Getting a tour of the dental practice also helps a patient understand the services that are provided, the staff working there, as well as the rules and regulations of the practice. Above all, dental practice tours usually help alleviate fear and anxiety. Dental anxiety and fear is a real thing a lot of people deal with, and it can be something that is overwhelming for the person going through it. As many as 35 million people are estimated to have dental fear which results in them not visiting dental practices.

The only way to maintain oral hygiene is by having regular and routine check-ups, and this also reduces complex and complicated treatments. If you ask your dentist or the front desk for a tour around the practice, they will allow this at all public places within the practice.

Thanks to new technology such as Google Street and Facebook 360, dental practices also offer a virtual tour of their offices and the surrounding so you can have a look and assess it before you come in for a visit or appointment.

More often than not, dental practices that feature the interior and exterior tours of their offices online have a higher chance of attracting potential patients and retaining them.

Are dentists allowed to give nutrition and health recommendations?

Dentists are allowed and should give nutrition and health recommendations just like any other medical practitioner. Except, a dentists' recommendation would be more focused on your teeth and what is recommended to maintain a good set of pearly whites.

The dentist will also give you recommendations based on your treatment. For example, if you recently had braces done on your teeth, the dentist is most likely going to advice that you eat soft food such as oatmeal or soup for the first few days/weeks as opposed to eating food items such as chicken and meat which would compromise the newly installed braces.

A dentist will also give you advice on eating healthily and cutting down your alcohol intake while carrying out routine checkups. A dentist's vantage point is perfect to pinpoint the health issues you have since they have direct access to your mouth. Poor oral health is a good indication that there are other health problems you may be having.

Do dentists usually offer warranties on their treatments?

It is a gray area when it comes to warranties on medical procedures and treatments. Usually, where the warranty is concerned is, it is usually related to the fixtures or components that are used in the patient.

Peace of mind is definitely important, and for Americans, insurance and protection plans contribute to dealing with half of this peace of mind when it comes to restorative, cosmetic and removable dental treatments.

To give you an idea, here is a quick summary of warranties that are usually offered by most dental practices:

- Crowns: 5-year warranty
- Dental implants: 20-year warranty
- Ceramic Veneers: 3-year free replacement warranty
- Bridges: 5-year warranty
- Root canal treatments: 5-year warranty.
- Fillings: 3-year warranty

Most practices around the country either offer or provide coverage to their patients that last about 1-year minimum to 6 years minimum. Patients are also given nationwide coverage which they would be able to use at any dentist or affiliated dental practice.

Coverage is usually the full original fee for the said treatment which also covers some lab costs and chair time. Ensure that your dentist provides a written policy of what is warranted and what is not. If your dental practice handles dental issues on a case-by-case basis, this is another red signal.

A written policy usually states the stand that the dentist takes in their work, the patient's responsibility as well as what the patient can expect in the event that there is an issue. If your dental practice does not have a written warranty, you can either use a different service or demand one.

Another thing to understand with your dental practice is how many redos they provide. This is great for your peace-of-mind, and if your dentist does give a few redos then this is something positive to note of their quality of work, and you can give them a five-star rating.

How can your dentist remove mercury silver fillings safely for you?

Firstly, let us agree that not all dentists are equal. One dental practice's procedure can be different from the way another dental office does it. Some steps could be similar, but depending on how invested the dentist is in getting a good job done, there may be differences in the ways of treatment. Also, the dental staffs' education and awareness is a crucial element especially when it comes to the relative toxic nature of commonly used tools.

Apart from the dentist, it is also the responsibility of the patient to educate themselves on the necessary protocols because this is an important health milestone. As a baseline, you want to minimize the risk of being poisoned during the procedure which is why educating yourself is important as well. It is for you to know if your dental team knows what they are doing and it is also so you do not do things that could increase potential risk.

So does the human body absorb mercury? The Journal of Oral Rehabilitation published a study in 2011 entitled 'Changes in health complaints after removal of amalgam fillings.' This study featured researchers testing the levels of mercury in urine and blood serum among the participants. Researchers did a test before and after the removal of mercury amalgam fillings.

According to the study, the scientists showed that mercury concentration in both urine and serum significantly reduced after the mercury amalgam was removed. When visiting your dental practice and speaking to your dentist about mercury amalgam removal, you should also ask the right questions to be absolutely certain that the dental team is equipped to help keep both the team and the patient is safe during this procedure.

What can you do as a patient before the amalgam removal procedure?

First, just make sure you schedule an appointment for this treatment at a calmer, reasonably free period in your schedule. This may not sound like it makes sense but try to get this done at a time that stress level is not high, such as when you are about to go on a holiday.

Your dental team will do whatever they can to keep exposure to mercury to the minimum but doing this treatment at a time that you are highly stressed may cause extra burden to your body. So do this when you are calm and reasonably free.

Second, you want to make sure detox glands and paths are functioning well. This is extremely crucial because we need our body to remove any mercury from our body. Our primary detox paths are our livers, bowels, kidneys, lungs and of course your skin. Here is a quick list of tips that you can get started on to prepare yourself beforehand:

- Stay hydrated.
- Eat foods that will support healthy bowel activity.
- Practice some deep breathing.
- If you have access to a sauna, use it.
- Take activated charcoal and a natural toxin-binder such as chlorella before visiting the dentist
- Increase vitamin B intake
- Do not take vitamin C in the morning before the procedure as it can disrupt anesthesia

These are just the simple things that you can do to

protect yourself and not jeopardize the possibility of increasing any risks or further exposure. Vitamin C is great to take after the procedure to encourage more detoxing and healing of the body. Most dental teams also provide vitamin C intravenous drip after the procedure.

How to protect yourself during the appointment?

Here is a list of procedures that dental practices normally use to ensure a safe and secure mercury amalgam removal. You can refer to this checklist with your dental team, or they might brief you about their own safety protocols beforehand:

- The room must be extremely ventilated with an air filtration system.
- Make sure that your face, neck, head, and chest are covered by a protective material.
- Your dental team will offer you a source of

fresh oxygen to breathe.

- A dental dam will be placed around the tooth that is being restored.

- A saliva suction device will be placed under the dam to suck up any vapor that leaks under the dam.

- A high volume vacuum will be used right near your mouth during the whole procedure.

- The dental team needs to use lots of cool water during the procedure. This helps keep the mercury amalgam cooler, thus reducing the vapor and help to gather and rid your mouth of any mercury particles from the removal process.

- At the end of the procedure, the dam is removed. Thereafter the patient will be asked to vigorously swish with some activated charcoal in water for a minute or two to gather and absorb any vapor that may be lingering in their mouth.

These are just some of the basics that the dental

practice will employ during this process. There are newer better refinements done to the safety protocols to ensure that safety is an optimum priority for both the patient and the dental team. Knowing these basics will definitely get you headed in the right direction.

What do you do after the procedure?

Keep your detoxing methods going on for the time limit that your dentist advise you. The best practice is to keep everything flowing well. There would be other strategies that you can check out online to ensure that any traces and particles of mercury are removed as well as with any heavy metals from your body.

How to find a dentist trained in safe protocols

One of the best ways or places to get proper and correct information is through the International

Academy of Oral Medicine and Toxicology (IAOMT) or the ADA, American Dental Association which can give you a full list of trained and certified dentists.

What is sedation dentistry?

One in three Americans suffers from dental anxiety, according to the American Dental Association. In America, fewer than 1% of dentists offer IV sedation because this requires special certification. Because of this, many patients are not aware that this sedation is possible.

Sedation dentistry refers to the administration of sedatives when there is absolutely no other way to cope with a patient who has severe dental anxiety. While there are many different types of sedation, the general resolution of using them is the same, which is the patient will only regain complete consciousness after the treatment has been completed. General anesthesia, as well as nitrous oxide, are among the two sedatives that are usually administered to both children as well as adults for treatment.

Nitrous oxide is usually known commercially as laughing gas. This gas is mild and analgesic and usually used by pediatric dentists. It is a safe combination of oxygen and gas which is inhaled via a nasal mask. The effect of this gas is within five to ten minutes. Nitrous oxide is never used as a general anesthetic in a dental office. This gas does not put a patient to sleep, rather it gives the patient a feel-good feeling which reduces their fear, apprehension, anxiety and pain sensation. It enables most people to relax as it provides a pleasant sensation.

General Anesthesia is usually administered for long and difficult procedures and especially when the dentist would require the patient to remain still. General anesthesia is a comfortable form of treatment in a controlled and safe environment for both adult and children.

Does your dentist provide flexible scheduling around work and school?

Between managing work responsibilities and attending events and activities and running errands, finding the time for dental check-ups would probably be the last thing on your mind. The problem that many people face is not giving dental care a priority. We rather choose drinks with friends over a dentist appointment. No matter how hectic your schedule is, regular dental cleanings are a must not only maintain a healthy smile but also ensure good oral health. Here are two ways you can ensure you secure a dentist appointment and stick to it:

Schedule your appointment either at the beginning or end of your day

When deciding on a dentist, one of the things to look into is ease of access, which means are they conveniently located at a place you can get to easily and if their hours can accommodate your schedule. Look at their schedule and see if they offer early morning or even late evening or weekend appointments? Do they have flexible opening and closing hours? For most people, afternoons are usually chaotic, and you're probably at work anyway at this time. If this is the case, you can make an appointment with a dentist that offer early morning appointments so you can get your regular checkup before heading to work. This is the same with evening appointments as well- you stop by the dentist for your appointment before you head home.

Look for a dentist with same-day appointments

Planning is always not the most ideal especially when your day isn't a routine one. Sometimes you need to stay back late at work or other times, you have an urgent project to rush, or your spouse or child is ill, and you need to attend to them. The most convenient form of appointments for someone with a busy schedule is to find a dentist that allows for same day appointments.

Most dental practices nowadays do not only offer same-day appointments for emergencies but also for regular appointments. Usually, dentists offering this service will schedule you in at the earliest available appointment slot before their actual appointments begin. This would help you from always canceling your dental appointments.

Cosmetic Dentistry

It is a valid question to ask about the difference between general and cosmetic dentistry because many people do not have a clear idea of what it makes the two different. In a nutshell, general dentistry focuses on the treatments and prevention of oral diseases and oral related problems whereas cosmetic dentistry deals with the aesthetic appearance of teeth.

To make it even more understandable, general dentistry deals with making your teeth feel better and cosmetic dentistry deals with making your teeth look better. Knowing the difference between these two types of dentistry can help you make informed decisions on which service of dentistry is right for you based on the issues you want to be rectified.

General Dentistry

General dentists usually deal with problems associated with oral discomfort and pain as well as oral hygiene. General dentists usually perform treatments such as filling cavities, tooth extractions, and root canals. General dentists also do tooth planning and scaling and also performs limited cosmetic procedures such as teeth whitening and bonding.

If you are looking to make your teeth look better, a cosmetic dentist can do that for you. They conduct treatments and procedures such as extensive teeth whitening, porcelain veneers, inlays and onlays, dentures, tooth colored fillings, fixed implants as well as smile makeovers.

While there are differences in the types of things cosmetic and general dentists, do, sometimes these two overlap as well. For example, if a patient has decaying tooth, then this tooth would need to be extracted to prevent the decay from spreading. This is usually done by a general dentist. However, the general dentist will probably recommend what cosmetic dentistry that can be done to improve the situation of having one tooth gone. This is usually taken up by a cosmetic dentist who will provide options for improving a patient's smile by either getting porcelain veneers.

Can teeth cleanings and exams be conducted by both General and Cosmetic Dentists?

Both cosmetic and general dentists go through the same training, but a cosmetic dentist would have had additional training and education. For example, a general dentist might conduct teeth whitening by removing stains from the teeth through scaling- this while great, doesn't really give you a Hollywood megawatt smile. If you go to a cosmetic dentist and request teeth whitening, you probably need your teeth to be cleaned first, then a more extensive whitening procedure takes place which usually involves laser whitening, a whitening solution, and the like. If you have a decayed tooth that needs repair, a general dentist will probably suggest extraction after doing some X-rays because their primary goal is prevention. If you go to a cosmetic dentist to obtain a more aesthetically appealing solution, the dentist will take x-rays prior to giving you options, extraction being the last of it.

Are prices different between General and Cosmetics Dentists when it comes to the same procedures?

Yes, there will be price variations from one dental provider to another depending on the procedures that are performed. Remember that not all dentists are created equal? Also, depending on the goals of the general dentist and the cosmetic dentist.

Which dentist would be best to replace a missing tooth?

When it comes to replacing a missing tooth, both types of dentists can do the replacement, and the most common treatment would be to use dental bridges. However, a general dentist will also refer patients to a cosmetic dentist to get a dental implant to replace a missing tooth.

Selecting an AACD specialist

More importantly, what is an AACD certified dentist? Founded in 1984, the American Academy of Cosmetic Dentistry has over 6,000 members and is the globe's largest and oldest dental organization. It has members in over 80 countries. This membership includes a vast variety of dental professionals such as reconstructive and cosmetic dentists, educators, researchers, dental laboratory technicians, students, dental assistants, and hygienists. The AACD was established to ensure, oversee and advocate excellence in cosmetic dentistry.

Not only do they champion the advancement of cosmetic dentistry, but the AACD also advocates the highest standards of patient care and ethical conduct through the administration of responsible esthetics. The professionals have membership in AACD have an obligation to display an interest in furthering education and to administer the latest advancements in cosmetic dental techniques, technology, and materials to their patients.

Why is an AACD accredited dentist beneficial?

As a member of the American Academy of Cosmetic Dentistry, education and training courses are offered to them on the latest techniques and procedures as well as products. The AACD also comes out with publications, provides workshops and lectures to members in order to ensure that these members continuously have opportunities to upskill and upgrade themselves.

The great thing about using a dentist that is accredited by the AACD is that they are always informed of market trends and learning the latest products and technology benefits that can be used safely on patients. Not only that their patients also receive up-to-date care.

To become accredited members, dentists have to go the extra mile to devote themselves to the qualities and standards established by the Academy.

What is the accreditation process to become members of the AACD?

Dentists who want to join the AACD have a rigorous process to go through. Candidates must completes a demanding clinical testing process which involves a high degree of both perseverance as well as commitment. A demanding clinical testing process is one of the exams that candidates must undertake and this itself demands perseverance and commitment.

There is a written examination and candidates must also provide five clinical cases as proof. Not only that, candidates must continue participating in classes as well as pass an oral examination. A dentist or lab technician that has been accredited, the dentist must at all times stay ahead with trends, new technology, and care.

Shopping around for dental prices

We do this for almost every imaginable thing on the planet- shop around for prices, compare side-by-side just so we know we are getting the most value for our money. Have you compared prices for dentistry though Here are some things to know when price shopping for your dentist:

Prices Vary Considerably

Most dentists do give a fair price, but sometimes it also depends on the dentist's location- are they in a central business district where prices of property are high? That would mean rental is high which would pass down to the dentist' fees to a patient. When checking for prices, also look for the location of the dental clinic.

Incomplete quotes

Make sure that whatever quotes you get cover not only what the dentist is expected to do but also the work that comes after it. Ask the front desk to specify what are you being billed for whether it is the cleaning, treatment, and aftercare or is it just the treatment and medication would be extra.

Low prices

Low prices do not necessarily mean bad service or bad dentistry. Most dentists give low prices for certain treatment as a way to attract patients especially if competition is strong. Most of these dental offices have figured out the game and instantly quote patients the complete pricing.

Be nice

When shopping for dental prices, it always works to your advantage if you ask nicely.

What about dental insurance?

Dental insurance usually comes in these three plans:

- Dental health maintenance organization (DHMO)
- Preferred provider organization (PPO)
- Indemnity Plan

Most of America's top 10 insurance companies all over DHMO and PPO plans and all but one provide indemnity plans too. Your selection of plans entirely depends on the dentists you choose and what you can and cannot afford to pay.

Dental Health Maintenance Organization (DHMO)

A DHMO is a plan that has lower-cost benefits and insurance. When a patient chooses this plan, this usually requires them to choose either one dentist or one dental facility as their primary care provider. Patients are only allowed to choose dentists that are listed in the in-network providers. A DHMO plan does not have any maximums or deductibles. Patients only pay a fixed dollar amount for the treatment that is covered by the plan, which is a copay. On the other hand, if the procedure is not covered by the copay, then the patient is responsible for all the costs involved. DHMO is the most cost-effective plan because it allows you to pay lower premiums and patients do not need to pay a deductible. However, in the event of a dental emergency, a patient could be stuck with the entire bill.

Preferred Provider Organization (PPO)

The PPO plan offers a patient the freedom to visit a licensed dentist of their choice to receive benefits, but patients get to enjoy a lower cost if they choose to visit a dentist within the in-network list. The services given here are based on a deductible amount as well as the coinsurance percentages on top of your additional monthly premiums. These plans actually cost a lot more in the long run compared to the DHMO plan. This is because of the higher premiums, but the good thing about it is that the PPO plans offer a more comprehensive and complete dental care coverage.

Indemnity

These kinds of plans offer the greatest choice for the dentist. As a patient, you can visit any dentist you want. The indemnity plan is similar with the PPO because patients also pay a deductible for each service, there is a fixed percentage of fees covered by the patient with the balance paid by the plan.

In the PPO plan, patients usually get a discount on procedures not covered by the plan. This is usually given by the providers of the plan. However, this option is not available in the indemnity plan so patients may end up paying more in addition to the monthly high premiums.

How these three plans work for you will depend on how many in-network providers the company that gives these insurance has your area. With the top 10 companies, they have over 100,000 network locations, and this gives potential dental patient's better and wider freedom of choice.

The first thing a patient needs to do is to inquire about network providers before deciding on a plan. Dental insurance providers usually have a plan for individuals, families, and couples.

Choosing dental insurance

Premiums for dental insurances cost less than health insurance, but there is a catch. While health insurance policies usually come with heavy premiums once you pay the deductible, insurance for dental have an annual limit coverage which is about $1000 to $1500 per year on top of the deductibles that is required which can range between $50 to $100.

Because of cost constraints that people face with dental insurance, it is not surprising that they delay treatment. Some put off treatment just because their insurance doesn't cover it or they have used up their maximum annual coverage, and the oral issue becomes even worse. So when choosing a dental insurance plan, here's what you can do and be on the lookout for:

Find out about Group Coverage

Most people get dental insurance benefits through the company that they work with or other kinds of group coverage programs such as the Affordable Care Act and the AARP or even public programs such as Medicaid, Tricare for the military and Children's Health Insurance Program for children. These kinds of plans are more affordable and individual insurance plans, and some may also come with better benefits. When it comes to an employer-sponsored plan, look at the details in the plan and decide whether the premiums are worth the money with your paycheck.

Check Individual Insurance Plans

Individual plans are both expensive and have limited benefits. Whether you are purchasing one for yourself or your family, individual policies often have waiting periods for major procedures. This is the same even if you are purchasing dental insurance because you are about to get new implants or new dentures or you have a treatment coming up. Insurers are well aware of this, which is why a waiting period of a year is included before you can start to enjoy the benefits of the policy. The best thing to do is to compare prices and benefits of policies from insurance company websites. Some, due to competitiveness offer shorter waiting periods.

Look at the Dentists listed in the Network

With indemnity insurance plans, patients get to use the dentist of their choice whereas using DHMO and PPO limit the choice to the dentists in-network. If you prefer using a dentist of your choice, then check with your insurance if this is allowed. PPO and HMO plans are great if you are comfortable using a new dentist that fits your needs. Speak to health professionals, your friends and neighbors to get some recommendation for a local dentist which they have found to be good then check your insurance plan to see if they accept that dentist. Keep a few choices on your list, so it is easier for you to settle with one.

Understand what the policy covers

It is extremely important to review the policies that you are considering purchasing. AARP Delta, for example, covers gum cleanings, restorations, oral surgery, denture repairs and root canals. However, patients need to wait until their second year of coverage to enjoy the benefits of these procedures and treatments. Even then, only 50% of the costs are covered.

If you need major dental work, then you would most likely need to pay a hefty share of the treatment cost. In both individual and group policies, benefits are limited, and it can vary according to insurance plans. Group plans also have waiting periods, albeit much shorter and they also pay a fraction of the cost of major treatments so this is something the patient needs to be aware of. Dental insurance coverage is great for preventative care such as the cleanings, dental x-rays, and checkups. Adults and children with dental benefits would be more inclined to visit the dentist and receive dental care, resulting in greater overall health.

Also, by purchasing dental insurance plans, you are more inclined to get preventative care and avoid more expensive procedures if oral issue gets worse. Be aware when purchasing individual dental insurance because major procedures may not be covered in the first year of your coverage. It is also worth setting some money aside monthly into a health savings account so that you are not caught off guard to pay for major treatment.

Dental tourism

The need for affordable dentistry is greater than ever especially with the rising cost of dentistry in America. Plenty of Americans, at least five million a year, are now looking into options of traveling abroad in search for better prices. Times are tough for everyone but if you are on the lookout for options overseas, what place is the best for dental tourism? Fortunately, options are aplenty on which countries you can go to get your tooth fixed. Dental patients can save up to 80% just by visiting a qualified dental clinic abroad. While most patients seek treatment in countries nearer to home, there is an increasing number who combine a dental trip together with a good vacation.

Here are some of the places you can check out to see most popular dental destinations and see how much you can save!

Why travel abroad for dental treatments?

Save Money: Money is definitely a factor, and you can save loads of money by just by choosing the right country, the right doctor and the right clinic for your dentistry needs. Most of the time, you can save between 70 to 80% for treatments abroad.

1. No Shortage of Options: No matter what country to ultimately decide on, there is no end to the options for treatment and subsequent care. Wherever you opt to go, there's no shortage of local options as well. In fact, even when you've settled on a country, you still plenty of options in choosing a clinic as well as a dentist. The bottom line is, the costs will differ. A country that has plenty of options is most likely the country with the best dental tourism.

2. Potential Savings: When you have your dental

implant operation in a different country other than your own, you can look forward to saving at least 90 percent of the cost if you are American. It is also due to the currency exchange rate with the country you are visiting.

3. Nearness: Ideally, you do not want to go too far to get a dental treatment done, even if you are looking for cheaper options. Most people in America seek treatments in Costa Rica and even Mexico. If you live in Europe for example, in the UK or in France, then your nearest destination would be in Poland or Hungary. If you are in Australia, your nearest destination would be the Philippines or Thailand.

Thailand

Typically, the prices in dental clinics average $746. Not only that, as an American, you can get access to world-class dentistry, but patients also have access to some of the largest and modern dental hospitals in the world. Thailand is one of the top ten places to go, and it is not secret! Most of Thailand's dentists are internationally trained, and the best part is, they work in a tropical paradise! Most frequent visitors to Thailand for dental tourism are Australians, Canadians, New Zealanders as well as Americans. Plenty of them come for a dental checkup or treatment but also for a holiday.

Mexico

A go-to dental tourism destination for Texans as well as for Californians is Mexico. Americans' who live at the country's south border prefer Mexico because it is a simple matter of driving there easily like driving from state to state albeit with the need to carry a passport. Americans that do not have the luxury of going to an exotic country like Thailand can easily opt to go to Mexico for not only excellent dental care but also dental care at a discounted price.

You can go to Mexico either by car or hop onto a plane and head over to resort towns such as Cancun, Puerto Vallarta as well as Cabo San Lucas for your treatments. Going to these places is akin to going to the Garden of Eden. These places are so beautiful you forget about your dental woes. Even if you do have dental anxiety, there is a likelihood that the symptoms might lessons because your mind feels like it is on holiday. On average, dental treatments in Mexico average around $750 for something like an implant surgery. The most common visitors to Mexico's dental services are Canadians and Americans.

Colombia

Colombia is another popular dental tourism hotspot and it is a huge appeal to dental tourists looking for a South American holiday. Not only is it great for dental tourism, it is also known for its American-trained dentists that have excellent Colombian hospitality but can also speak fluent English. Many dentists in

Colombia are not only trained in America but speak fluent English due to the influx of Canadian and American tourists coming over to seek dental treatments, implants, care, and checkups.

On average, dental treatments cost a mere $650 which is why Colombia, specifically Bogota is a viable candidate for the best city and country for dental tourism on top of being America's answer to Europe's dental bargains from Spain. Accommodations in Colombia may be a little on the high end, but it is all worth it with American-grade dentistry.

The 10 Questions to Ask Your Dentist

A reliable and knowledgeable dentist is needed for anyone, especially if optimum oral health is a priority for you. Dentists are not hard to find but it is important to find someone that can understand your dental needs as well as your preferences. Prioritizing your comfort and dental needs should come above monetary gains.

If you are in the midst of looking for a dentist, there are some essential questions that you can ask during your first visit which would help you ascertain the dentist's integrity and credibility. It will also help you decide if you would like to go to the same dentist or not.

1.   What is my overall health status?

This is actually one of the first few things that the dentist should tell you because this is what they would need to look into when checking your teeth. Understanding the health status your teeth and mouth are at that very moment helps them determine what procedures or treatments are needed, if need be. It will also help you, as the patient understand how good or bad your oral habits are.

2. Is there anything about my oral health that I should tell my general doctor?

Oral health is a big indicator of your overall health. Your mouth, teeth and tongue can give pretty good indication of what's happening in your body. Asking this question to your dentist also helps you gauge how receptive your dentist is to answering questions and also how accommodating they are in ensuring your overall health.

3. What can I do to improve my oral health? What can you do to help me improve my oral health?

Oral health works both ways. The patient needs to do a few things on their own to maintain oral health and the dentist helps the patient get to the oral health that they need. As a patient, understanding what your dentist can do for you helps in maintaining a good set of teeth and gums and it also gives you a better understanding of oral hygiene. Be aware of dentists that give you a long line of treatments and procedures.

4. How do you keep up with the latest dental science?

Asking this question helps the patient estimate the level of expertise. Knowing your dentist keeps up to date with dental technology and science would ultimately give you peace of mind as you know your dentist if giving you the best treatment there is.

5. How often do you want me to visit you for periodic check-ups?

Knowing how often you are required to visit your dentist for check-ups is part of patient-dentist relationship. It helps the dentist understand your needs and availability and it also helps you understand the dentist's treatment times and opening hours.

6. Is there anything that the dentist needs to know from the patient's family doctor?

Sudden complications in your mouth could be a result of medications that you are currently taking and this can cause some changes in your body and also any treatments that are administered by the dentist.

7. What preventive techniques to you recommend based on the current status of my oral health?

The answer to this question pretty much depends on the state of your oral health. Again, be wary of the number of treatments or procedures that the dentist is recommending you do. If this happens, it is always good to get a second opinion from another dentist.

8. Do you specialized on a specific field of dentistry?

A great way to get to know your dentist! Understanding their expertise enables you to stay informed and even recommend friends and family to this particular dentist.

9. Would you be able to provide me with an estimated cost of the treatment you're recommending?

A dentist should be able to give you the full cost of your treatment and any other potential additional treatments, especially if the procedure or treatment is a general or standard one. This helps you know if you are financially capable of meeting the budget and if the dentist's charges are something that you can afford.

10. What are your payment options?

Knowing the various payment options helps you when you need to undergo an extensive treatment. It helps you plan and budget wisely.

Conclusion

I hope you've enjoyed this book and that you now feel adequately prepared to choose a dentist.

You should now be armed with all the know;edge you need to get the best value and quality you can afford when it comes to dental care for you and your family.

If you enjoyed this book, I'd appreciate it if you left a review on Amazon

Thanks,

John Mitchsell

www.ingramcontent.com/pod-product-compliance
Lightning Source LLC
Chambersburg PA
CBHW071225220526
45468CB00002B/730